T0129837

STROKE, HAVE YOU HAD YOURS YET?

John Lipsett
CD Airforce Chief Warrant Officer

Order this book online at www.trafford.com
or email orders@trafford.com

Most Trafford titles are also available at major online book retailers.

Printed in Victoria, BC, Canada.

ISBN: 978-1-4269-2948-9

Library of Congress Control Number:

*Our mission is to efficiently provide the world's finest, most comprehensive
book publishing service, enabling every author to experience success.
To find out how to publish your book, your way, and have it available
worldwide, visit us online at www.trafford.com*

Trafford rev. 4/15/2010

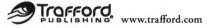 www.trafford.com

North America & international
toll-free: 1 888 232 4444 (USA & Canada)
phone: 250 383 6864 ♦ fax: 812 355 4082

Ageing process! Say what?

Was this my first Stroke? I can now be almost sure that mini strokes or warning signs were apparent months before, however attributed it to the ageing process and a blatant disregarded for what my body was trying to explain. Now the term, months prior to the main event, is meant to be eighty-four to ninety in total. If any of these signs sound familiar, there is good reason to have them checked out by a competent Physician.

To my signs, high blood pressure, at first was not considered but it should not be excluded. Having been put on medication some years prior, one learns that the medication does regulate the pressure to a point, however, pressure surges are still there and the older we get, the more important it is that we learn what causes these spikes and try to avoid those situations. Some of the following signs can be matched with high blood pressure and maybe even stroke.

On occasion one would feel a temporary loss of balance, not to be confused with a dizzy spell, while standing and/or putting on a sock. Realignment of the foot on the bed/chair or sitting down plus an effort in deeper concentration would remedy this temporary situation most times. Another symptom was the blurring of vision, mostly in the left eye. These events, would come and go occasionally but were more likely attributed to poor glasses, eye strain etc. Numbness of various areas of the body, in my case it started with the fingers and face. Sitting at the dinner table on at least a half dozen occasions, my wife explained that there was a small bit of food on my left cheek, this was a surprise as nothing was apparent or felt by myself. Upon removing the food particle, it was noticed that an area of numbness about the size of a dime was present at that location but disappeared a short time later only to return.

Good old ageing process again? I don't think so. Other areas were experienced around the nose, upper cheek and neck, never at the same time and not consistently enough to arouse a real concern. Finger numbness was attributed to freezing of the hands some years before. The left leg had twinges now and again, where the feeling left various areas and was replaced with a cold numbing sensation which would last for short periods of time. Now, to this point one would think that there is enough evidence listed that medical advice should be sought and it was. The reporting to the newly acquired family physician was met with this response, "You are growing older and have reached an age where you must expect these sorts of things" .which could be interpreted as *"all part of the ageing process"*.

What else could be wrong and why do we have all those blood tests yearly? Many articles have been written about strokes and the benefit of certain drugs as possible prevention should one take coated ASA on a daily basis? I do now! Hindsight is the better of the two and I will never know if starting to take the drug when my wife wanted me to and she started, would have prevented what has happened? One other thing that the professionals found out about my post stroke condition is that the vitamin B and Folic acid levels were dangerously low in fact non-existent. This information was collected and further studies of other patients concluded a direct relationship between low levels or lack of these two minerals could be one contributing factor to strokes.

Relocating to Ottawa, corrected a lot of things however, it didn't completely solve the phobia of seeking medical advice when things aren't right. As the non activity of retirement caused a weight gain a self impose diet shed the unwanted layers plus drained the body of a lot of its strength, something I would pay dearly for in the future. A serious bladder infection worsened to the point where by the time medical assistance was sought the bladder was periodically malfunctioning and had grown to about the size of a professional football. Prescribed high powered antibiotics immediately went to work on the infection but voiding of the blood filled urine remained a question and would last for many more days. Apart from this, previous Ultrasonic testing of the prostate indicated an enlargement, not in the medals category but large enough to possibly impede the voiding process. Of course, I didn't want to admit that the stream had lessened somewhat, well OK, I couldn't write my name in the snow anymore and this concerned me. *Trouble in River City,* you say! Well, I guess. Now from a time line stand point, this took us from early November to the 3 of December 2000. *My stroke day!*

Stroke day- 3 December 2000

The day progressed as usual, running to the bathroom every hour due to the severe bladder infection. Now, after 14 consecutive days and nights of endless running produced one tired soul. After brunch, it was decided to rest for awhile on the living room sofa. Right on the one hour schedule an urge for the bathroom stop returned. Rising to the occasion was no problem but while heading to the stairs the strides were seemingly exaggerated and the arms produced the largest of arcs as a speed skater in full flight but this was only an illusion as my wife witnessed the whole exercise and saw nothing wrong. It was like gliding through a medium. At the bottom of the stairs all returned to what was perceived as normal in my mind and never occurred again.

The bathroom mission was accomplished and a lay down, this time on the upstairs bed produced another hour of rest. The next trip to the bathroom was a totally different story and one I hope will never be repeated. From the toilet, rising again to the standing position, now this statement maybe foreign to some however, having four of the fairer sex in our house for a number of years, one adjusted his bathroom habits immediately after the first occurrence, well maybe the second, to avoid those midnight screams, "*Who left the toilet seat up!*" "*Help*" or "*Mommy, I'm stuck*", "*Help*" So again, rising to the standing position met with a moment of unawareness, the only time during the entire episode that this was experienced or at least I thought so until future event unfolded. As was evident by the subsequent bruising of the arm, head and side I had uncontrollably fell toward our Roman bath tub and with a glancing blow finally crashing to the floor but regaining consciousness at that point once again. Hearing these unusual sounds my wife inquired if everything was all right to which I replied, "No", "I think something is terribly wrong". This brought her upstairs and with one look at me she dialled 911 for medical assistance.

Trying to assess what was happening while waiting for the paramedics to arrive established very little but panic. The right side of my body had next to no movement. The left side, especially the arm and leg were lifeless and felt like weights which anchored me to the floor. Trying to position oneself to a more comfortable state was impossible in fact nothing was possible except the mind was going a mile a minute with all sorts of unanswerable questions. Once the medics arrived, they pressed into action, taking vitals, asking many questions and reassuring me that all would be OK. Quickly, it was determined that I was having a stroke and was prepared and ready to go for a ride to the hospital that would accept me. *Accept me! You have to be kidding, aren't you? This is Canada where hospitalization is assured?*

One of the questions that was asked during the initial process was if I had any preference as to what hospital I was taken to, I indicated that it would be nice to go to the one that my family doctor was associated with and was told they would try their best but at the moment that hospital wasn't accepting patients. *Whoa!* One of the largest area hospitals isn't accepting patients? Not even stroke victims? I couldn't believe what I was hearing or didn't want to believe what I just heard but was reassured by the paramedic that this could change at any point along the way. Now my mind really went into high gear and I was glad that the vitals had already been taken as the BP had probably reached the maximum or beyond calculations. As all hospitals were west of our house the odds could be 50/50 but not necessary in my favour. My understanding at that point was that once an area hospital accepted a patient they have until a certain road turn-off point to change their mind. Now their mind can only be changed if another area hospital closer becomes available, the first could say *OK*, you take him. Now when you think about this it isn't really all that bad should you be so lucky to be in an ambulance but what happens if you do not have the same radio contact and are travelling in a private vehicle? In retrospect, one should be thankful that there is more than one hospital in the area and at this point we hadn't even left the house yet so my wife would be told which hospital we were headed for and would be called if anything changed.

Montfort here we come, maybe?

The hospital site was established shortly after leaving home and the ride to the hospital was pretty uneventful, however the pace soon quickened upon arrival at the Montfort Emergency Dept. I have never been given this much attention before in my entire life time. Transferred to a hospital type stretcher and wheeled to and fro from this testing machine to that. First the CT scan, Doppler and back to emergency and finally into a bigger more comfortable bed. The Neurologist who had been directing this episode from the very first approached my bed side to introduce himself, ask a few questions, check some of my reflects and explained the different avenues that could be explored to ease the situation. He explained the "*Clot Buster*" its actions etc. and indicated that because we were still within the time frame required and that it was a clot that was causing all this havoc, recommended its use. Accepting, the clot buster was administered and the waiting game began to see what effect it would have. The next major event was the installation of a catheter upon my request where after, I heard the nurse; we have a real gusher here, standby for the overflow and measurement. 1 litre, 2 litres and finally, voiding is slowing, must be coming towards the end. What a relief! To both my bladder and the thirst buds. Where' the water jug? This cat is drier than a wooden hen. As the clot buster went to work a significant major event was the change in the left limbs, suddenly, I regained control and some movement was accomplished. Raising the arm and waving the hand at the doctor and nurses met with smiles of approval. Raising of the left leg and wiggling of the foot met with the same approval. This was however, to be short lived and the best kept secret within that room was the fact that I was listed as "*Critical*" even with these movements.

As the afternoon turned into evening and night, my world quickly became more concentrated, to an area between my face and the ceiling. Staff, now only faces, would regularly enter my world, these short visits disturbed the much needed rest that was required and in my mind deemed to be unnecessary. The hospital staff knew differently however as these checks were to determine my state and any changes in it. The paralysis slowly but steadily returned until my left side was completely paralysed and my right side started showing similar signs. My head internally, felt swollen but without pain. Speech became slurred and I found it harder to pronounce the words. Most evident was the swelling of the inside of the mouth. The tongue became a regular target of the teeth. The inner cheek also would not escape the Pearlies as more than just a few times a gash would appear. All was very annoying to say the least and caused various amounts of pain. Drifting off to what I thought was sleep my world as I knew it came to an end sometime later that evening.

A transfer from Emergency to the Intensive Care Unit occurred during the next few hours, this relocation took place without my knowledge but my family informed me as to how the drama unfolded after I regained my senses.

For the next few days it was still a wait and see situation. Before leaving Emergency I did again respond once more to the doctor, whose voice I seemed to be tuned into and the only one that was now recognizable. Remembering him explaining that the clot was in an inoperable position had been partially dissolved however; it had a long tail which had embedded itself further into that portion of the brain. Medication such as regular ASA would be administered and hopefully this tail would go completely but only time would tell.

Again, drifting back to the unknown I suppose my condition could have been upgraded or downgraded at any point but I was unaware of any changes for the better or worse. As it turned out on the seventh day I awoke from this nightmarish state in a regular hospital room on the second floor with the neurologist giving me one more examination at 5:30 AM before going off to another assignment outside the hospital. He kept repeating the time and apologizing for being so early and hoped that I would understand. He talked about the swellings, the droopy face, left side paralysis, plus the problems I would encounter with the eating of solid food. His last comment cautioned me about sitting up for the first time then suddenly he was gone. Was I dreaming or did this conversation really take place?

Waking up some time later I could see what seemed to be a glowing light exhibiting a beautiful blue hue slowly drifting across the ceiling then disappearing only to return moments later. Could this be the light at the end of the tunnel those with near death experiences talked about? Shear panic and fear was the order of the moment plus another concern came to mind, where had my family gone? Had they been here? Droopy face, what droopy face? Be careful upon sitting up, why? And the list of questions was never ending and seemingly nobody around to answer them. Facial twitches turned into body tremors, fretting turned to outright FEAR, Was this going to be as good as it gets for the rest of my days? Oh God! I prayed, Please help me!

My prayer was interrupted momentarily by a nurse who said "Welcome back" and inquired if everything was OK? Now on the *emotional roller coaster* that would be the norm for sometime to come I pleaded, with teary eyes not realizing that my speech was garbled beyond recognition to a lay person, *"Have my wife and family been here though this ordeal"*? *"How long have I been here"*? The questions were endless. She assured me that all had been here and that my wife would be back this afternoon. They had sent her home to get some much needed rest as my condition had improved somewhat?

The awakening

Waking up to what some would say was a stroke induced comma to find your body completely paralyzed except for your tongue which felt like it was three times the size of a Beaver's tail and twice as woody, a dull ache which engulfed everything from the neck up plus eye lids that seemed prepositioned at half mast and a mind that was going a mile a minute. Now the left side paralysis was understood but what about the right side? Was it being sympathetic to the left side or was it shear fright that caused the motionless state? Would time tell?

The nurse, who caught the first signs of my re-born existence, was an expert in garbled, slurred and intermittent speech, although I couldn't tell much difference. She answered the pressing questions and told me that she was not an angel and what I thought was a near death experience seeing the blue hue of light on the ceiling was nothing more than the projection of the hospital worker's endless stream of car headlights coming through the window as they arrived for work. At this point I asked for some water. Bringing the glass and straw she positioned my head to the right and instructed me that she would place the straw well into my mouth and then

I was to try and suck the water through the straw. After many attempts some actually went down my throat but most came out the left side of my mouth. *Droopy mouth you say*!

What has improved? "Well, your urine from your bladder infection is certainly a much lighter pink, which is a good sign and the doctor says that the stroke has gone as far as it's going to go". "Now", "please try and get some sleep and I will wake you for breakfast". My mind now had started to clear to a point where things, faces and all that were viewed was becoming clearer and more familiar. Once I was told that my wife and family had been there and she was returning, certain calmness entered my body and I again turned to prayer. "Thank you Lord, for my precious wife and family" Upon completing this prayer, another story filled my mind and that was the story called *"Footprints in the Sand"*. It was a story where Jesus was explaining to an individual that the two footprints in the sand were of themselves as they walked through life. When the foot prints became only one set the individual asked. "Why did you leave me Lord"? Jesus replied "I didn't leave you; those were the times that I carried you". At this point I was so hoping that there was only one set of footprints in the sand in my life's story as I was so hoping that Jesus was now carrying me and somehow, I'm sure he was as I drifted off into a deep more restful sleep.

The day did not start off with breakfast but a bed bath headed the list. This probably wasn't my first but it was the first that I was aware of. After the announcement of the bed bath I couldn't stop thinking of a story my mother-in-law use to tell of her bath experience in the hospital. She told the tale that the nurse would wash down as far as possible and then up as far as possible but she would wash possible. This wasn't the case here as possible had to be checked and cleaned daily by the hospital staff due to the catheter and the attached outside plumbing, so professional cleansing was automatic. Sure felt good but I missed the running water of the shower.

Breakfast was accomplished by raising the head of the bed up and placing pillows either side of my head and again the tilt was to the right. Hoping for eggs, bacon and hash browns; I had to settle for liquids, liquids and more liquids. At one point I thought a little voice in my stomach was saying, "Hey up there"! "No more fluids, we need lumps down here". With a lot of slurping, gagging and coughing what didn't run down my chest via the droopy lip ended up where it was intended. These experiences were also the first time I could fully assess the lack of mobility within my body. Turning over from back to front or from side to side could only be done by the nurses. All which added to the complete feeling of helplessness and at that point I wondered how does one get up out of bed, move around etc., but was to scared to ask.

Recovering at Montfort

The time line at this point was murky at best, however, the events are forever etched in my memory. The next was like an old time reunion. To see your precious wife followed close behind her by your eldest daughter; that is a sight to behold! It didn't matter that the eye contact told the story of what they were seeing even though they tried so hard to hide it. The important thing to me was that I could recognize them as to whom they were for the first time in what seemed like a life time. I should tell you that there was a complete turn around in my emotional state due to the stroke. Prior to, I found it very difficult to display emotions and crying was out of the question except for a couple of occasions, family deaths and births.

Mixed emotions, there might have been, but I was the happiest person in the hospital at that moment. Hugs, kisses and tears gave way to more hugs, kisses and tears until all had their wits about them enough to talk. This is probably the hardest time to get through because there really isn't any answers to the enormous amount of questions everyone had but I found out later that they were better informed than I. You see, our family doctor had visited the Emergency prior to my entering the comatose state and I remember thanking her for all she did for my family and I, plus I hoped that she would continue doctoring forever. She then spent a lot of time with my family and kept them abreast of the changes. It was her, bless her heart, which gave them the hope that I would someday, down the road, get better.

The afternoon sped by quickly, we also discussed the pros and cons of going to a private room which was available, all agreed and the transfer took place immediately. That same day, the swelling of my throat and tongue started to slowly disappear plus I detected the sporadic involuntary movement of the fingers of my right hand. This turned out to be the start of better things to come. After an examination, the swallow test proved that the inner things were returning to normal in some of the upper extremities. Great news! Solid food could be attempted some day, maybe, hopefully with a lot of luck.

The first breakfast of liquid was certainly an experience. Thanks to the professional nursing staff, what could have been a disaster was avoided. Now a practical exercise is far easier to understand than a simple explanation, right? So the next time you go for breakfast, with everything on the table, to make it easier for you, try only using one hand for everything. Just before you start eating, place the pointer finger of the other hand in the corner of your mouth and pull down your lip so that the bottom teeth are showing. Now you are ready, enjoy! You will find it a little easier, as we haven't ask you to bite your tongue and cheek a few times just to get the true and the complete feeling.

The right arm and hand started to respond and within a short period of time I could move them with some difficulty and the main objective being to reach my mouth. Once this was accomplished solid food was the topic of the day. Much easier said then done, luckily for me all the food was taken out of its wrapper and placed in the appropriate containers. Jam was put on the bread after the butter and so on. All juice, milk containers were opened and positioned on the right side of the tray. A few timely tips such as placing the straw well back into your mouth before sucking, avoid placing food to close to the front of your mouth, try to place it well back on the right side, take real small bites and chew real slowly. Lastly came the bib and it was funny, I never even asked why. The meal was without mishap and necessity being the mother of invention, I did quite well. Drooling was the order of the day however, one soon learned if you turn your head a bit to the right side after putting something in your mouth it helps to keep it contained. Drinking from a glass or cup was impossible. Having consumed enough to sustain this rather large frame, the nurse congratulated me for doing such a good job and proceeded to take away the tray and clean me up.

Scary moments and movements

Life in the new room was more quiet but the regular routine remained the same, At bedtime the nurses would ask me which side I preferred to sleep on, then after turning me they would pack pillows between myself and the bed rails to retain the desired position. Meals posed the same problems but I was becoming handier at helping the nurse open the packets using my teeth and eating with one hand although muscle weakness hampered many attempts at either.

The Physiotherapists arrived and outlined the program of working together starting with balance. After other brief explanations as to how we were going to proceed down went the side rail of the bed. Within seconds I found myself sitting on the side of the bed being held by the therapists. Now, the question was posed, "Can you sit up straight by yourself"? My reply, "well, if my head can be stabilized", and with that they assured me that I would not fall and immediately released their grasps. All went well for about two seconds when my head flopped to the left, followed by my body. Caught and repositioned, the next fall site was behind me which again indicated how much the stroke had affected all my muscular functions. Neck manipulations were carried out to imitate muscle memory and to strengthen them. One of my do-it-yourself exercises while lying down was to repeat all neck movements several times going as far as I could each and every way. At first, movements were almost imaginary with little or no movement at all but over time things started to change with rotation and nodding first accomplished.

The sessions that followed worked on controlled side to side, back to front movements to strengthen the trunk and butt muscles and to regain some resemblance of balance. The forward movement proved to be the scariest as you could see where and what you were going to hit should someone miss catching you. Now, when you have a little control you have a little say in what is going to happen but when you have no control it is devastating to say the least. One must master the art of sitting because it is not only a requirement but the basic position where most everything begins. Never thought of that before, but it certainly spurred me on. It was also the first indication as to the toughness and the enormous length of the road to recovery that I thought I realized before, little did I know.

The question of getting out of bed and moving around came one afternoon as the therapist entered my room pushing what seemed to be a crane. After the impending exercise was explained a blue harness was placed around and under me and attached to a hook on the crane. With the flip of a switch the purring started, a sound I learned to despise, then up I went lifted off the bed, the crane was then pulled out until I cleared the bed. A wheelchair arrived with the third therapist and I was lowered into it. Still having little but some control of my neck and butt muscles, I was packed in with pillows and then straps were positioned and buckled to secure and maintain the sitting position. This new found sense of freedom was most inviting and a feeling of renewed hope prevailed. To this end, I fought continuously flexing one cheek and then the other. Back and forth while propped in bed or in the wheelchair more than just a few times, I had to call the nurse to retrieve the pillows off the floor. Persistence paid off, within a few days I was ready to take this chair for a spin or at least I thought I was ready.

Learning the technique required in controlling the chair with a paralyzed right arm and hand, plus a right leg with similar characteristics without crashing into the walls etc. proved to be another pebble along the rocky road of life which had turned into a huge bolder. Trial and error was the order of the day and by night times I had most moves under control and was doing baby wheelies around the room, but still to frighten to venture into the hallways. Like a kid with a new toy, I didn't want to give it up but the repeated day activities and my weakened state quickly caught up with me to the point of shear exhaustion.

The physiotherapy continued but not in my room. Loaded into the wheelchair and pushed by a porter, we arrived at a gym where specialized exercise equipment was housed. This was to be my place of workouts, stretches and tugs, groans and moans, for the rest of my stay at Montfort.

A peek see, we'll see

The jury is still out on what really caused the stroke but the best guess from the specialists was that a clot from the bladder infection made its way up to my brain and caused the mayhem. The urologist, on a visit to my room said, "That the bladder infection was rapidly clearing up and that a look inside should be done to ensure everything was OK". Speaking of phobias, this was grade "A." Seeing the look of terror or panic he methodically explained the procedure done through the urethra and it would confirm the presence of any growths, obstructions or damage etc., which may be present. His mannerisms, like our family doctor, soon dispelled any fear for the moment one might have and he left with a positive confirmation. I think?

Positive until a form was delivered for me to sign granting clearance and turning over parts of my body that they deemed necessary to remove, well not really, it allowed them to keep and do whatever they wanted with any biopsy material that was obtained during the scope exercise. Standard procedure the nurses said, "So please sign here", which I did. Now the signature probably wouldn't stand up in court as it looked more like a hen scratch than a signature. No sooner was the ink dried on the paper and I was transferred to an examination table and was being scooted down the hall. Overhead signs were flashing by as quickly as I could read them and it wasn't until I read Operating room 1, that I really started to pay attention. Gliding right by produced a short lived sigh of relief as we stopped under a sign Operating room 2 and was left alone there to fret. A nurse finally approached looking for the sign form, retrieved it and said, "I will be back in a few minutes". Soon the doors of Operating room 2 opened and there stood the doctor awaiting his patient. The nurse reappeared, rolled me in and commenced to prepare the sight for the examination.

Questions were warranted as the doctor started explaining what he was going to do as soon as I entered the operating room. Having left my hearing aides in the night table, yes that too, was a hindrance as both ears were damaged prior from working in the Air force around aircraft for thirty-seven years, I did not hear the preamble but felt a tug on my bladder and an "Oops, best we let the air out of the little bulb that holds the catheter in there before trying to remove it". Then holding up both the tube and scope he informs me that fact the scope was just a little bigger than what was up there already. Surveying both I wanted to scream, *"You're going to shove that big thing up where"*?

Almost like the dentist saying the tooth is out, after you ask him when he is going to pull it. All went smooth and soon I was heading back to my room. At the elevator I said that I hoped that lunch was still being served as I would hate to miss it. A voice from behind me remarked, plain to see you haven't talked to the physiologist yet.

Another medical professional visited that afternoon; it was the doctor from the Rehabilitation placement Organization. He was there to evaluate my condition

21

and recommend placement or not, to one of the Ottawa Rehabilitation Hospitals. Placement didn't mean that you automatically went to a facility of choice but would possibly be put on a waiting list for the first available bed in any of the facilities. His interview started out with the usual tap on the limbs for reflex responses and the first question was, what date is it today? Do you know where you are, in what hospital? What are your aspirations for the coming months? Now the first question was the hardest. Upon retirement the first thing you get rid of is your watch, second the calendar. I was retired for over ten years so how was I supposed to know? I did know that Christmas was coming soon, though my grandchildren. The last question was the easiest, I wanted to get better, drive our van again to take my wife and family out to dinner and get back out on the golf course. He thought those were pretty tall aspirations as he looked over this lifeless body just having been put back to bed for an afternoon crew rest, but I assured him that if I was lucky enough to get into a good rehab. facility I would show him what could be done. He wished me luck in all my endeavours and said that before he left that day, placement for an institution would be finalized or not.

Shasta knew, transferred too.

There has been mention of my wife, daughters and granddaughters visiting and a combination of them along with our son-in-laws made for many most pleasant times and helped with a bad situation. I also hoped to see our furry person, Shasta, a Keeshond by breed. We found out that this could only be accomplished with us going down to one of the entrances were she could be brought to that location. This meeting was important to me but at the same time I dreaded what it might bring. Being raised on the farm with all kinds of animals, you soon learn or suspect that they are special and we are now learning just how special dogs are and what they can detect in humans. Our first meeting was arranged and my worst thoughts came true. Shasta looked at me, heard my voice but her response was completely negative. She would normally be all over me but not this time. What did she see that made her respond this way? That question we will never know the answer to but it certainly bothered me and would until our next meeting. To satisfy myself for the present, I made up the excuse that the surroundings were new and that she was frightened by the doors that kept opening and closing but I knew I was only kidding myself. She somehow knew something was terribly wrong with Dad.

The exercises continued, I learned to move the affected arm with the good one. Had I been scheduled for a longer period, more sophisticated equipped might have been use for my legs but this was not to be due to the timing, however, what was received was greatly appreciated.

Medically, to date, the swelling in the old cranium continued to subside, biting of the tongue or cheek only happened occasionally but I was still in partial denial, thinking like a person that never experienced a stroke or forgetting that I had one. Wake-up day was soon coming!

Being catheterized played no part in the transfer, the outdoor plumbing would be tagging along as it did on the wheelchair and hopefully it wouldn't get caught up on anything.

The word came late in the afternoon that the next day between 10:00 and 1200 noon I should be ready to go. My family gathered up the personal belongings that evening and placed most of it in the van as only one bag was permitted to accompany me in the ambulance.

Leaving Montfort Hospital was an exciting experience with mixed emotions, it marked the next stage in the recovery and I was beginning to look forward to the change. Not because I didn't like the way I was treated there, as the treatment was nothing but First Class.

It was time to get on with the more intensive therapy in one of the facilities better equipped for patients in my condition that everyone was telling me about. The place that I was destined to go didn't seem to make a difference as all in the area had good reputations and people who were experts in their field. The send off was most pleasant with only one small delay which allowed for lunch to be consumed and more time for my family to get to the hospital. The time line became clearer now. Stroke day was 3 Dec, and Montfort stay was through to the 18th so in a private room for 8 days, the remaining 7 days was spent in Emergency and the ICU.

For those who know me, you have probably realized that I am writing this account well after the fact, from notes mentally scripted and jotted down throughout the timeframe. On 3 Dec. 2010 it was the 10th year anniversary of my stroke but it seems at times, like yesterday as I go through and describe each event. Each page contains the important events and each page has its emotional highs and lows. Many tears have been shed thus far explaining these accounts and more are likely but it is producing a type of closure for me with the hopes that someone out there also gets some comfort that they are not alone while going through a similar situation.. The next hardest part is the typing, all has been accomplish with the use of one hand, and one finger which could only indicate it's a true labour of love which I must continue until all the story is told. St. Vincent is waiting.

St Vincent Rehabilitation Hospital

We were met at the main door by three of the nursing staff from ward 1D who welcomed us with open arms and explained the admittance procedure. My wife was sent to do some administrative functions and as we rolled down the hall to my room, many questions were answered. One I asked was if this old body could be fixed; one of the staff said, "Why for sure Sir", "Miracles do happen at St. Vincent". For those who have read my poem by the same name, you now, know the rest of the story. If by chance you haven't, read on, it is part of this my story.

Via a three person transfer I was placed in my new bed and told that a temporary wheelchair would be made available until mine could be measured and fitted. Should I feel up to it, I could be placed in the wheelchair for the remainder of the day, including supper time or I could stay in bed? Should I want to get up, dressing would be a must as this was a rehab. Hospital and everyone gets dressed. My decision was to remain in bed for the rest of the day so as to get use to my new room and the sites and sounds of my new surroundings. Plus, my family needed time to unpack and redecorate the room with all the get well wishes etc., especially the drawings our grandchildren and class mates had made. I did however, want to have supper and get up for breakfast in the morning. Eating supper was accomplished with my families help and it seemed that more was heading for my stomach rather than down my chest from the droopy mouth. This revelation called for a "Cry-for-happy" event by all present.

The rooms were not that large for two beds and a cabinet for each patient but they were positioned to give us maximum space. Each room had a large window, a common wash area plus two doors, one leading to a shared bathroom and the other to the main hall. All patients had their own private telephones and of course call buzzers to the nurses station should a nurse be needed. Intercoms to the station were also available. The closets for clothes were built in, each one with ample space for all the required clothes and anything else you might want to store temporarily. Above the sink there was a shelf large enough to house two TV s complete with the sound wiring back to each bed. This allowed for earphones so that one patient could watch TV without disturbing the other. Of course, each bed space was curtained for patient privacy.

The nurses thought that it was probably the correct decision on my part to stay in bed as a number of people would be in to see me including a hospital doctor and therapists. Within a very few minutes the doctor arrived and briefly outlined the program and the tests that would be performed. She explained the requirement for blood tests and other tests i.e. TB, to ensure that I hadn't brought anything with me. They would be started after fasting, probably as early as tomorrow morning. Other tests and EKG would be scheduled, as to not to interfere with my therapy, within the next few days. After hammering at my reflex points and observing the reaction, asking numerous questions and yes, two were, do you know where you are?

And what date is it today? She turned the floor over to the physiotherapist and left after indicating she would be checking up on me each and every morning for the duration of my stay.

The Therapist outlined her part of the program which would not be started until a complete assessment of my condition was established. Tests mainly would include, among others, mobility analysis and sensitivity tests, beginning in the morning by her and other therapist from Occupational Therapy Department (OT).

The rest of the afternoon and evening was left for rest, relaxation and a wonderful visit of my wife and family. We discussed many things. One of which included the paperwork to obtain permission for Shasta, our furry person, to enter the hospital as it was discovered that the hospital staff welcomed pets and were well aware of their therapeutic value. My family seeing that I was well looked after, left for home for a well deserved rest from this event filled day.

Prior to bedtime the nurses brought me a light snack and some apple juice then at the appointed time again as they did in Montfort, asked me which side I would like to sleep on. They turned me and packed the required numbers of pillows to hold me there. Sleep came quickly and was a deep sleep until early morning my bed light came on and a voice said, "I'm here to take your blood!" All I could see was what seemed to be an 8 inch syringe bearing down on me. Was I dreaming?

Another awakening

Morning arrived with a second bright light flash, this time from the main ceiling light and a cheerful "Good Morning Sir!" "We are going to give you a bed bath, help you get dressed and help you into your wheelchair for breakfast OK"? "Sounds great to me"! To satisfy my earlier encounter or lack there of, I checked my arms for bandages and sure enough one was present on my right arm so it was no dream I had given a donation.

All other events were accomplished with swiftness and professionalism; soon I was being hoisted via sling into the temporary wheelchair. For breakfast I had a choice of eating in my room, or out in the hall with the other patients, due to the lack of proper dinning facilities. "Oh, let's go out in the hall so that I can meet others like myself". A *bad decision on my part!* "Nurse, please may I eat in my room". Being very obliging she rolled me and my breakfast tray back into the room, not saying a word, but the shoulder taps said exactly what she felt and was very comforting for the moment.

The next few minutes were used to collect ones thoughts. What did I actually see out in the hall? People slumped over in their wheelchairs, some quietly sobbing in anguish and despair. They were repeatedly sat upright and consoled by a passing nurse, bibs on all patients, some of which were covered with the current breakfast or slobbers and left/right side limbs that lay dormant unable to move. *Is this me? Do I?* With that analysis I wheeled myself over to the mirror and the *Realization hit me like a ten ton truck*!

At this point I knew I was indeed, one of them however, luckier than most, I was spared the full extent of the lasting facial paralysis, the cranial swelling had reached a point of reversal where thinking was much clearer and I had already been taught to sit upright. I too, was motivated into getting better by my loving family and friends plus my faith in God to give me the strength to overcome this earthly affliction was ever on my mind. Could it be that the people out in the hallway were less fortunate? The coming days and weeks would tell and answer these questions.

The physiotherapy evaluation was scheduled for 11:00 am and was the only thing listed on my events calendar. Reporting to the gym thanks to the hospital porter, still shaken from the earlier experience, offered some relief or at least it put my mind on other things. The first evaluation was hopeless. As they went down their list they finally came upon one that I could do. Sit in an upright position without support, well almost no support. These results, however, were over shadowed by the ones I failed and the emotional rollercoaster had once again kicked in big time. Depressed, I guess, but I managed to hide some of it, I think. My main fear at this point was that I may not be able to do what was required in physiotherapy and therefore my future was full of uncertainty again.

Exhausted and breaking for lunch, I was requested to return as soon as possible so that the other tests could be done. These continued tests included largely sensitivity. While blind folded the therapists would brush areas of my body with cloth, feather or touch with warm or cold test tubes to see if the feeling was there. My task was to determine which area they touched and to identify that area or if it was hot or cold. I did much better in these exercises which turned out to be a plus for me; however, in my mind I had one big unanswered question. Did I do well enough to qualify for the rehabilitation program or was my brain still too scrambled and body to weak to realize or do what the requirements demanded to proceed?

Returning to my room I was greeted by a lab technician who informed me that he would do an EKG immediately. Being again, hoisted back into bed, the EKG was done with only one rerun. Of course, as soon a problem is detected and another run is required, you automatically think that there is a real problem with your heart and nothing to do with the instrumentation. Asking the lab tech doesn't help much as you can never get an answer that you can fully accept. For example, at my request he simply said "the spikes are there, some going up and some going down which is a good sign", immediately thereafter he left the room.

That being done the nurse paid me a visit and we discussed the possibility of getting rid of the catheter collector bag that I haven't really said very little about but it was always a problem. Each time I was put in the wheelchair, this sac had to be unhooked from under the bed and reposition under the chair and the hose positioned so that it wasn't hanging to be run over or stepped on. She indicated that now that physiotherapy was scheduled, they would look into ordering a leg bag which should arrive within a day or two and it would be fitted at the earliest possible time. This should be more convenient and allow greater mobility all around. (Physiotherapy was scheduled) *This was music to my ears*, I had done well enough or at least was now accepted into the program.

Worlds turned upside down

With the evaluations completed, the physiotherapists could now do an analysis of the requirements and map out a strategy as to which areas needed what therapy during which time. We discussed her approach which also provided a way of getting to know each other and finally parted with the understanding that she was the expert and whatever plan she developed it would be followed and completed to its fullest. A real cake walk! *Wrong again!*

One of her comment or questions didn't really register at the time but would come up later as I lay in bed waiting for the sandman to arrive. The question, how are your wife and family coping with the circumstances of your stroke? To this point, with my brain still active but not firing on all cylinders, everything was about *Me, I, and My.* It was about *Me,* I had the stroke which left *Me* in this condition and *My* world was turned upside down! As I lay there the question haunted me more and more until I finally and suddenly realized that my wife and families world was also turned upside down and I was not the only one affected. My mind was now working over time; my wife had her drivers licence and drove but was satisfied to let me do most of it for years. This meant that she was forced, in the dead of winter, to drive not only to visit the hospital but to survive. Now the head of the household with no one to confer with placed an extra burden on her already laden shoulders. She sat alone hour after hour pondering our future, not knowing what was in store, however, not once lost her faith that everything was going to turn out alright. Her sleepless nights and worrisome days started to take its toll but I was too blind to see until after that night. I got little sleep wondering how I could help. I'm afraid that was as far as I got because my brain had lost its ability to organize or formulate a plan however, the important thing was it changed my attitude and got my mind off of *Me* which I found out later was an important step to recovery. It was also discovered, that to have a loving family to partake in your step by step rehabilitation, giving the reassurance that daily progress was being made was a priceless benefit.

At exactly 6:14 am the next morning I was awakened by someone with a flash light trying to check my identification bracelet. "Good Morning", this little soft low voice said, "I am here to take some blood for the lab, hope you don't mind". With that she proceeded and was gone in a flash. She was so good at what she was doing that when I awoke at the regular time, I again, had to check to see if I had given blood or was I dreaming.

Apart from these special wake ups, the wake up routine had become just that, but things would soon change as my personal notice board became more crowded. It had already been changed to include appointments for Occupational Therapy (OT) Monday and Thursday at 11:00 am or sooner and Physiotherapy daily at 1:00 pm.

Physiotherapy

Preceding with her plan of action my therapist methodically applied her developed techniques to my limbs commencing with my affected leg. Stretching, flexing and massage to reduce the tone plus re-establish the memory loss and strength became the order of the day. Countless hours would follow with me wondering how she could maintain this pace especially when the initial applications produce seemingly limited or no results evident to me. This should have been very discouraging but not to her, she carried on like the professional she was only transmitting encouragement as she worked. With the initial applications completed I would then be turned over to a technician who administered the repetitions prescribed by the therapist only to have my therapist go on to the next patient.

By this time sitting had become almost common place and standing the next order of business for without it the harness and crane would not disappear or be replaced with a one, two or three person transfer. Of course to be standing you have to get there via some mode or other. Concentrating on my leg strength and accomplishing the same, my therapist then taught me how to get from the sitting position to standing tall. Her instructions were to lean forward using my leg muscles to raise my butt off the bench until finding a comfortable stable bent over position was reached, whereas the straightening of the trunk could then be done until the standing tall position was achieved. Scary or what, but she assured me that should things go wrong under no circumstances would any harm come to me. Having full confidence in those words the attempt was made but resulted with my returning to the bench unsure of my leg strength. Further attempts with a lot of prompting proved successful thus establishing another milestone in recovery second only to the first steps that would follow a few days later.

Apart from the countless hours of hands-on therapy other means to strengthen my body were employed. The therapy technician would place and strap me on the tilting table and supervise the leg exercises that were to be done. These proved to be very difficult and taxing but combined with the other mechanical devises were worth every effort as permission soon came from my therapist that a two person transfer was now permissible then that soon changed to a one person transfer terminating with under close supervision. Other milestones accomplished and a true testament to the labour of love displayed by my therapists and her technician.

Throughout my therapy the ritis boys repeatedly tried to disrupt my progress and arth was the worst. One amazing fact was that the arthritis in my affected areas seemed to lay dormant while the non-effected limbs continued to progress but at a slower pace. On numerous occasions upon completion of my physiotherapy the technician would place hot packs around and over my shoulders and arms to sooth the beast and invariably I would go to directly to dreamland only to wake myself up by my own snoring to the amusement of all the gym inhabitants.

When the weekends came all therapy ceased and the halls became quieter due to some advanced patients going home for a visit and other being discharged. To the patients that remained in house the hours dragged out and some wondered why these two days were wasted. At first, I too, questioned the fact but not for long. As soon as the therapy started on a regular basis one suddenly realized what the weekend was for, rest and relaxation so our bodies could heal. Not that we were hurt at anytime but the awaked muscles required time to get use to the repeated moving, flexing and the demand placed upon them. This healing process would be repeated day in and day out and a nights rest didn't seem enough at any time so the weekends became haloed time not to be rearranged in any way.

My weekend afternoons and evenings until bedtime, were the most pleasant as this is when my wife and most times, other members of the family or friends would arrive. As I got better even on weekdays we would sometimes wait for the evening meal trays to arrive and proceed to the cafeteria to eat together. A lot of times the tray was exchanged for a pizza, sub or the cafeteria special. Not that the hospital food wasn't good! Well! A change was always welcomed and a 1200 calorie, no salt, no sugar diet was in no way good for this 214 pounder.

You want me to build what?

The fast approaching Christmas holidays seemed to amplify the sense of urgency to get better faster. My therapist's plan for recovery was a testament to her professionalism and worked like a charm, I had already made huge strides in muscle movement and toning. Standing was achieved and became common place. The transfer harness and crane was dispensed with and replaced with a two person transfer.

For my bladder infection, the attached outdoor plumbing was replaced with a leg bag which proved to be less than perfect. On two occasions a warm sensation was felt in my right shoe. "Oh no"! "We have a problem nurse, a leak has been detected". Soon after the second episode a waist bag replaced the leg bag which proved to be the best of all. It was however, to be short lived as the infection was on its last legs and removal of the catheter and freedom from the bags was coming soon. *Wrong again!*

The Occupational Therapy (OT) department actions were initiated soon after arrival and in concert with everything else. Their instruction and help included helping with and showing how to get washed and dressed from a wheelchair using only one hand. These techniques proved to be a real asset to my recovery. They were also present during my bathing in the bath tub and subsequent trips to the shower stall when the time came for that exercise to be allowed. Oh, how good it felt! The only drawback was the placing of the harness and the hoisting in and out of the tub. This, for the moment, brought back memories of past events and was looked upon as a regression which no stroke survivor wants to ever experience.

Other contact with OT included upper body therapy mainly with my left arm being put through the range of movements plus further exercises for hand to eye coordination to name a few. Another task that was presented but not accepted by me was the in house building of a bird house. To qualify why I rejected this exercise and at this point my mind justified the refusal, I had worked on aircraft in the Air force for some thirty-seven years plus in the Non-destructive Testing field, we dealt with the Nuclear Industry developing inspection techniques for reactor fuel rods. You want me to build what? How about an Aircraft or Nuclear Reactor? Of course the answer was no, there seemed to be a shortage of parts available for either. All therapists must have patience and mine certainly did. She put it down to the fact that I was just not ready for such tasking and never again broached the subject. Her analysis being correct, other exercises were initiated to achieve similar results.

Next came the showering, this exercise had to be done alone with the therapist standing on guard outside the shower in case of an emergency. Sitting on a shower bench provided a sense of real freedom and progression. Once completed, one felt another hurdle had just been cleared, so bring on the next challenge!

It would soon arrive with the changing of the guard in Physiotherapy. My regular therapist had booked Christmas holidays off to return home for a family Christmas which was well deserved. My new therapist proved at once to be another true professional and my progression continued at a fairly rapid pace. Dwelling on stair climbing as she knew our house was a three level which we did not want to move from unless absolutely necessary. In the gym the stairs included four steps up and down. Having completed an exercise with ease with them prompted a bigger challenge. Transporting me in my wheelchair to the hospital stairs going to the next level she left me to contemplate my next move but instructed me to remain seated until she got back as she was called to the phone.

Viewing those 23 cement and steel stairs reminded me of a story about these two Maritimers (Mike and Joe) that decide to go west and get a job driving truck through the mountains from Edmonton to Vancouver. Once there, the prospective employer explained that they would be a team, while one was driving the other would be sleeping in the crew cab and they would be on the road 24/7. To judge their experience the employer asked Mike if he was driving in the winter months and came over the top of this mountain road and seen a huge pile up down at the bottom of this steep hill, which brakes would he apply. Mike said "Why the trailer brakes" "OK in the same situation, the trailer started to slide and you realized that the road was covered with ice, what would you do"? After a long pause Mike said, "I would wake up Joe". "You would wake up Joe, whatever for"? Mike replied, "Cause Joe never seen a big accident like this before". My accident would be tumbling down these stairs which of course was never to be as my therapist knew I could do it and she would be with me all the way to ensure success. It was her way in showing me that with guidance and self confidence I could accomplish more things should I put my mind to it and she was again right.

Merry Christmas and
Happy New Year

Christmas in the hospital has to be one of the loneliest places on earth. The regular staff is away or at home with their families. All patients that could travel were gone and the decorations that were hung did little to cheer us up. My roommate being one of the luckier ones had gone for Christmas Eve and Christmas day to his daughter's place which allowed my family more room to congregate. The weekend routine prevailed with one slight change; we were allowed to sleep in an extra hour. The silence was deafening for the rest of the morning but things did get better as the few families arrived. Children running up and down the hall were music to our ears and on occasion one would pop their head in and tell us what Santa brought them. My family arrived each carrying loads of goodies some baked some bought but nobody cared from where it came the important thing to me was it was there to be consumed. Sure glad the dietician was on holiday also as her motto was, if you put something in your mouth and it tastes good, spit it out! Only kidding! But don't you just hate those thin people.

Now at a normal Christmas at home when opening presents one would think about how one would use the gift or I will sure get some good wear out of this piece of clothing. These thoughts after the stroke were changed to I wonder if I will ever get a chance to use or wear these presents. Our grandchildren spent a lot of time amusing themselves by pushing each other or driving themselves up and down the hall way in Grumpies wheelchair. Now this is not a typing error Grumpy was the name given to me by my oldest granddaughter; you see, when she was learning to talk, she would go to say Grampy but it would always come out Grumpy. That is my story and I'm sticking with it. Even in her school where I took both grandchildren and picked them up every day I became known as Grumpy Gramps, Their principal, on one of his visits to the hospital brought me a framed get well wish addressed to Grumpy which I will cherish forever. All in all we had a wonderful day and I was thankful that my family made it that way. New Years was somewhat similar however, more patients stayed in so that meant more families arrive which turned out to be an event filled day which we were glad for the solitude of the late evening.

The New Year continued with more challenges, my therapist fresh off of a Cape Breton home holiday stayed the course first set out by her, she would work desperately to get the limbs moving to their fullest then would turn me over to a technician to do the repeat exercises before she went on to the next patient. Hours spent on the standing or exercising on the tilt table was hard at first but as time went by more time could be endured which indicated the strength was returning. Eventually more walking was necessary to coordinate those leg muscles and improve balance. Armed with a pole in the right hand and my therapist on the left side we slowly ventured out of the gym gaining ground on each attempt until the entire length of the hall was covered. I will never forget the look on my wife's face when I walked into my room were she was waiting for the scheduled family conference to begin. It was priceless. Lots of "cry for happy" followed.

The family conference was a meeting to identify the progress or lack of for one Johnny boy. It was attended by my doctor, a nurse, my physiotherapist and my Occupational therapist and of course my wife and myself. The doctor started with her comments indication that the Vitamin B and Folic acid levels were now at the desired levels and that the medication would be continued for the rest of my stay. She also mentioned that the diet was working and I was losing weight at the recommended weekly levels plus the bladder infection was in its last stages. My physiotherapist had nothing but praise for my efforts and I for hers. However, the Occupational therapist said," John was a bad boy because he refused to build a birdhouse as part of his therapy". She also indicated that further down the road they would introduce me to the kitchen and meal preparation. With this my wife thought that this would be unnecessary as my mother had taught me as a boy, how to do everything in the house from cooking, baking to clothes washing, pressing etc. So the kitchen duties were scratched. Other things that were discussed were a pending home visit and possible weekend visits at home for me.

Special visitations

My appointment calendar kept on growing as the days past; apart from the physiotherapy and OT sessions there was a trip to the Speech therapist where it was determined at that visit that speech wasn't a problem. The physiologist too dismissed me after his session or I should say we parted with the mutual understanding that further consultations were not needed. Our visit included the old standard question and answer session. "Do you know where you are"? Answer: "In St. Vincent". "Do you know what time it is"? Answer: "Well it must be around 14:00 hours, as that is when I was scheduled to see you". "Do you know what day it is"? Answer: "Not off hand, but it should be close to Monday". I could see by his facial expressions that he wasn't satisfied with the answers so I decided to run this summation by him. "Sir", "I retired some eight years ago and at that time I put my watch in the top drawer of the dresser and removed the calendars from the wall". "Until I came here I got up when it was light outside and went to bed when it got dark". "I ate when I got hungry and that's pretty much it".

The Recreational Therapist also visited, inviting my wife and I to an outing at a wheelchair accessible restaurant with other patients and their families. This we declined thinking that I just wasn't ready but in hind sight I now wish we had of gone.

The hospital Pharmacist paid a visit checking on my medications and explaining the patient meds program which would be initiated sometime in the coming weeks.

Not regularly scheduled were the frequent visits by one of the Sisters of Charity of Ottawa. Knowing that I was not of her faith, she introduced herself and immediately said "She was not there to convert me but to comfort and encourage me during my stay at the hospital". A very pleasant lady who had a way of making everything seem better and less complicated, her repeated encouragements and discussions assisted greatly in my mental healing process.

I would be remiss if I didn't mention another regular daytime visitor, our youngest daughter. She would leave her office some eight blocks away, regardless of the weather and take her lunch hour with dear ole Dad. Picking up some low calorie items on the way we would share them out of sight of the diet police. The remaining time would be spent rubbing my affected foot while silently asking the good Lord to please return the life to it. Her husband, our son-in-law made every effort to visit and came in at suppertime bringing pizza or subs during a two week training session he was attending across the street. Sometimes his visits coincided with my wife and oldest daughter's but the days they couldn't make it due to the weather he filled in for them.

Mentioned before, our furry person Shasta, (a Keeshond) was another true family member and not seeing her left a huge void in my heart. The word came through that the hospital administration had approved her visitors pass and she would be allowed in for visits. I had mixed emotions about her reaction because of the results of our Montfort meeting still lingered in my mind. Would she still act strangely towards me? Normally a very protective canine especially where her family was concerned, we always kept a rather tight rein on her so as to not allow any undo aggressiveness. Anticipating the arrival, I ventured out in the hallway but kept a fair distance from the main door. Two or three patients were between us. As she arrived in the ward, to my surprise, Shasta, in an extremely cautious mode approached the first patient, sniffed the wheelchair then the outstretched hand of the patient, something that was completely foreign to her. Normally she would keep her distance unless told otherwise by one of us. The next patient the routine was the same, she even allowed the lady to pet and scratch her. Watching this I could not hold back any longer so called her name. With that her ears went from the half mast to the full up position, knowing the voice she headed straight toward me and ended halfway on my lap, at least the front 40 of her 80 pounds were there. The tail was rotating like the blades on a helicopter and my face received its second cleaning of the day. I do believe she was smiling the rest of the evening and demanded that she be placed on my bed with me beside her. Normally we would play rough neck but not tonight nor on any subsequent visits. She sensed my condition so a gentler exchange prevailed. Even when the nurses came close Shasta would watch very carefully but not offer as much as a low growl. What brought this 180 degree turn around could be a mystery to a lot of people but not to us. We knew she was intelligent and talented so we talked to her as if a person right from puppy hood; her responses amazed everyone who met her even the most skeptical. Shasta made a lot of friends in the hospital, staff and patients alike, what made her so special in the eyes of some was she always had time to say hello or goodbye, sometime going right into the patient's room to do it.

A matter of trust.

You might wonder why one would write about the following and include it in a stroke recovery story but I promised myself that I would include all traumatic events. Traumatic, in this case was for a person whose body on numerous occasions, was being invaded by unfamiliar objects. We could say also attributable to his loss of dignity. I now have some idea what ladies go through when their feet are in the stirrups on an examining table.

The doctor arrived early in the morning doing her rounds and told me that the bladder infection had disappeared completely so now the catheter could be removed. This would be done as soon as the head nurse got a minute. Identifying my joy to a couple of people one said, "Why on earth would you want to get rid of that"? "Just think you can drink all you want and never have to get up anytime to go to the bathroom". "That is true but you don't have to wear one!" was my reply. The head nurse and I finally got together and the extra baggage was removed to my relief. Now I could do all those things people were suppose to do and a sense of total freedom prevailed, but not for long.

The doctor returned to explain the forthcoming procedure for retraining the bladder. The months of being hooked up caused the bladder to forget what to do or became lazy. Voiding would be a problem, but normally only for a short time. She explained that we would keep track of the amount voided and even provided a log to be filled in each time. Now to show the bladder what it is suppose to be doing I would be checked every four hours via a meter and should an excessive amount be recorded I would be cauterized to empty the bladder. The next few days were a nightmare! Try getting your proper rest, doing your therapy etc. when you are awakened every four hours. Even therapy took second place to the organ retraining. Starting to look and feel like a zombie, I requested an extension, especially at night. The doctor agreed and the schedule was moved to every six hours. I mentioned the meter for measuring bladder content. The one that was there never seemed to work properly, giving erratic readings or no readings at all. It was replaced a couple of times, of course with a faulty meter, better use the catheter, got to be sure!

One would hope that you could trust your nurses at all times, right? Well the procedure for catheterization initially called for some lubricating/desensitizing gel to be placed on the catheter before insertion. The tube was carefully removed from its protective wrap and placed on a sterile pad. Then the cap was removed from the gel tube, some squeezed out or appeared to be squeezed out and applied to the entire length of the tube ensuring every inch was covered. This exercise in all cases was completed, going over the tube two or three times for whose benefit, the patient's of course. What a show!

They talked about going home for a home inspection and for the weekend. This was totally dependent on my bladder returning to the proper or normal operation, unless someone in our family would do the catheter task or if I could do it myself. Well, call me chicken. Fortunate for me my wife volunteered to be trained by a nurse. The same procedure was followed and she passed with me not feeling a thing. Armed with enough catheters for the weekend, she made sure all was done by the book. Now one should be able to trust his own wife right?

The catheterization continued for longer than expected; however, I was starting to get frequent urges especially at night. With the sense of feeling gone one couldn't tell if venting into the jug really occurred. Once the urge had subsided the jug would be shaken to reveal its contents. Many disappointing tries lead to further frustrations until one early morning things felt different. "By Gosh", "I think I did it" Still not allowed out of bed on my own I waited for the nurse and asked him to confirm what was in the jug. He took it to the washroom and came out with a big smile and announced that a miracle had happen. Oh what a relief, good bye catheter. *Wrong again!*

The doctor explained in the morning that now that I was venting on my own, they would have to make sure the bladder was draining to an acceptable level somewhere in the neighborhood of 90 milliliters. The process continued until the second weekend at home which was two weeks down the road. Finally, all returned to normal. Now back to the aforementioned trust; seems that the application of the gel was for show only. Checking my top dresser drawer the tube provided for home had never been opened. After much questioning my wife finally admitted that as long as the patient thought it was covered with gel that was all that mattered and it worked. Can anyone be trusted these days?

Survivor to survivor

As a people watcher many things happened that most were unaware of, but to me the events were both disheartening and joyful. When a patient's brain failed to give them the ability to respond to the instructions of the therapist, this was disheartening. For these many hours of various states of depression consumed their day and night. Family members were beside themselves sometimes blaming the hospital staff, the program and the therapists for their relative's state. This couldn't be further from the truth as I witnessed the repeated attempts by all staff members to try to hit a chord with all patients so that recovery could proceed. These attempts in most cases were successful but on occasion failure was imminent as the brain was in control and wouldn't respond.

These patients bothered me to no end and I often wondered what would be their final outcome. One such case I would stop in the hallway or visit their room and try to talk to them. Patient to patient had some effect but in no way could I take credit for the turn around. I did witness their first step but lost track due to my release. Would the system let them fall through the cracks? To my relief I experienced a patient who was removed due to the lack of response but returned some weeks later to therapy when the response became active.

For those who could apply themselves and learn to do what was required to get better that was joyful. Unable to do the movements required for life and after hours of therapy that first step was monumental. Only problem is that you wanted to run with the wind however, your therapist knew better and would caution you to take it easy and slow down. The number of times I heard, "stand tall", "taller", "and taller", would knock your socks off but would grin and bare it as I knew I would be three inches taller than when I was admitted. Would you believe one inch.

Another event that turned out joyful happened one evening after I had said goodbye to my family and was returning to my room. I witnessed a patient standing by the nurses station all dressed in her street clothes with her suitcase beside her. Starting up a conversation I was informed that as soon as their family arrived it was homeward bound for her. From the outside you wouldn't think this was a stroke victim, her abilities to walk etc. were not impaired and even talking to her you could be fooled. Not knowing the doctor and nurse had spent a lot of time trying to get her away from the idea of going home I proceeded to question her motives. After explaining that she thought home was where she should be because she was well again, I agreed to disagree and told her what I would do so that my family would not worry if in her situation.

The conversation continued for another thirty or so minutes when I returned to my room to go to bed thinking that my efforts had fallen on deaf ears. Sometime thereafter the nurse entered my room and asked "what I had said to her". "Just talked patient to patient why"? "Well, whatever you talked about convinced her to stay; she is now unpacked and sleeping in her bed". "It's wonderful as the doctor and I talked until we were blue in the face and couldn't change her mind". "You did", "so there must be something to this patient to patient thing that we have experienced from time to time".

Another situation occurred while travelling in the hall, approached by a doctor he informed me that he had a bone to pick. Upon entering one of his patient's rooms he witnessed his patient distraught and tears rolling down his face, Confused, the patient asked "why his demeanor had changed so much, was he going crazy"? The doctor explained using textbook medical terms that it was the effects of the stroke and not him that was to blame for his change in emotions and him being put on the emotional roller coaster. Being unsympathetic and still confused with the answer the doctor further explained the situation in layman's terms which now seemed to be somewhat understood. Then looking the doctor straight in the eyes he said, "Well doc, you must be right because John Lipsett said the same thing and he's been there and done that". The doctor's conclusion, "keep up the good work John"!

These and other similar events, some involving family members, convinced me that a lot could be communicated all for the betterment of everyone concerned. Not knowing that forums were available for such an exchange, I promised the Good Lord that when not if but when I got better and was able to chauffer myself around I would return to the stroke ward and try my best to encourage the patients to continue their therapy and try to help them better understand their situation.

My days of in-patient therapy were quickly coming to an end; then I was offered another two weeks. Checking with my family all thought this would be a great idea and very beneficial so the extension was accepted. It proved to be a good decision as further improvements followed and ones even I could see. Looking back I often wondered how one got through this ordeal and my theory has concluded that the Good Lord orchestrated the whole affair and made sure all was well. The other two parts of the triangle were the beautiful people, some assigned to renew this body and my loving family who stood by me all the way.

First trip home

Prior to home visitations the patient has to be able to manage his or her own medications should they be taking any and most are on something. The program starts out with the patient requesting the meds in the hospital from the nursing staff at the appropriate times. Once passing this test the pharmacist provides the patient with a week's supply of medication which was kept in the locked drawer of the bedside cabinet. A key was assigned to the patient for their use only and is worn around their neck so to be with them at all times. This became a symbol as it indicated responsibility and a milestone in recovery. Periodically the nursing staff would request that you show them the medication tray so they could determine that all was going well and that no meds were missed.

Our Occupational Therapist made all the arrangements for the house inspection visit. It was required so that things that may be a problem for me could be identified and changed or removed. Signing me out with my meds in tow, oh yes, don't forget the catheters, our trip commenced. After a horrific ride in the taxi the snowy driveway became the first hazard encountered. Treading with caution and assist by the therapist we made out alright and entered the house. The two porch steps didn't pose a problem neither did the two steps to the living room from the vestibule. The only difference was the living room was carpeted which most know is a nightmare to stroke survivors. Seems your affected foot always gets caught up in the fiber. I had been warned about this many times so was prepared to put in an extras effort to make sure my left foot was raised enough as not to scuff. The therapist inspection of the main floor living area including the kitchen and a powder room, all were clear of any hazards. Next the upstairs with six steps to a landing, two more to another landing and finally five to the upper level. Railings were only on the right side going up so given I could get up the stairs, how about coming down? They say a picture is worth a thousand words so a demonstration should work better. Given the courage by my physiotherapist I ascended the stairs with ease. Getting to the top I rested while the upstairs inspection was completed. Some recommendations included a hand bar for the shower to assist my getting up off the shower stool that had been recommend and purchased a short time before. Also a toilet extension could be installed should I find the seat to low and had trouble getting off it.

Ready to go downstairs I was requested to show how I could manage. Turning around I held on to the railing with my good hand and went down backwards one step at a time. To everyone's amazement I did better going down than coming up but an important observation was identified, that was what would I do in the case of a fire? I suggested that if that was the case and I had to get down in a hurry, my butt may get some rug burn. The stairway discussion was completed with the recommendation that we get railings installed on the other side as well. This was done and my trips up and down got back to normal, up forward, down forward with absolutely no problems. The same situation was present for going down into the Recreation room so railings were also installed on those stairs. Satisfied that the place was reasonably safe the Occupational therapist bid goodbye and I proceeded to explore all areas with exception of the bathroom where this nightmare happened. We had the usual family visitations as it was sort of a novelty to have Dad back home, if only for a short time.

One problem that arose after going to bed was the fact that I had lost so much weight, 214 to 165 lbs, that my wife had to shake the sheets to find me. Other than that all was well, our bed, our home, our family and our furry person, who was also elated to see me and remained at my side most of the weekend. Things were heading in the right direction thanks to the physiotherapists and all their hard work. The rest of the weekend sped by all too quickly; however, I was thankful for the opportunity to be with my family and exercise my new found skills plus the meals were delicious. When Sunday evening rolled around I knew I must return to my home away from home for more rehabilitation knowing it would soon be time for me to return for good. The trip was another major factor in my recovery; it proved my therapists had done an excellent job in preparing me for my new life. Thanks to them my life was back on track and they helped to make me what I am today.

The family

Much can, has and should been said about the staff both in and associated with ward 1D, the first contact each weekday morning was the ward clerk who quietly placed the patient's food menu on their bedside table the be filled out sometime that day. She would speak only if you were awake, her cheerful greeting would be followed with positive comments for the day ahead. The choices on the menu were normally threefold but as found out early, you could substitute the odd entry as long as it fell within your dietary schedule. My favorite was changing the dessert for ice cream.

Next to enter your room was the nursing or Occupational Therapy staff, depending on what stage you were at in your rehabilitation. If you had been shown how to wash and get dressed or if it was your turn for a bath or shower the Occupational therapists or staff normally looked after your needs. Always gentle and companionate they would repeat the instructions or exercise until the patient was successful doing it on their own. Socks were difficult to get on with just one good arm/hand so a plastic tool was made that could open the sock and enable the patient to slip it over their toes. Buttons also posed many problems so continued practice with their guidance always proved successful.

The nursing staff was forever around to add a helping hand and did on a continued basis. They were the guarding angels ensuring the patient's privacy and safety throughout the entire in-room events. On completion of the washing/dressing they would deliver the breakfast tray opening those pesky boxes and lids on plastic containers, just to name a few of their duties. Without their continued guidance and assistance the preceding would be disastrous and in some cases impossible.

Physiotherapists and technicians, those other dedicated professionals who spend countless hours working those affected limbs with sometimes limited or no response but this doesn't deter their efforts. They are truly the miracle workers.

The domestic personnel would often enter the room going quietly about their duties. They seemed, as everyone in the family did, to have an eye for patient improvements and would pass on the compliments when engaged in conversation.

As a tribute and sincere thanks to these wonderful people and my family and friends I wrote the following poem. Being unfamiliar with rhyme, it was apparent that I had some help from above as it was written in two twenty minute sessions. Its impact has been more than positive as family members have broken down while reading it and some staff has said that if they have a bad day a reading makes them feel better. God bless all!

"Miracles DO happen at St.Vincent"

High above the LeBreton Flats,
Not far from the river's shore
God had erected a stately place
Where his work would continue for evermore
Since its inception, many have entered its doors
And no, it is not a coincidence
You see, Miracles DO happen at St.Vincent.
The staff in this place, their dedication is outstanding
As is their caring and understanding
One would wonder with such a collection,
How did they get there from every direction?
These people of quality;
Was it by luck, by chance or have they been sent
Remember, Miracles DO happen at St.Vincent.

From the front lines a personal perspective,
Witnessing the actions became most exciting and never
deceptive
I watched the tears of anguish and despair turn to "cry-
for- happy" laughter
When a three person lift became a one person transfer.

When those affected limbs began to move and went
from straight to bent
You knew, Miracles DO happen at St. Vincent.
I too, was terribly challenged, far beyond
comprehension,
But let's no forget the power of prayer and divine
intervention
This body graduated from being lifted about to standing
tall,
To short assisted jaunts up and down the hall
By the grace of God the paralysis slowly went
Yet again, Miracles DO happen at St. Vincent.

Thank you Dear God for the strength to overcome this
earthly affliction
Thank you for my precious wife, family, friends and
their understanding and affection.
Thank you for those with conviction, who gave us the
encouragement, hope
And were the first to proclaim that,
Miracles Do happen at St. Vincent.

By John Lipsett St. Vincent Ward 1D
18 December 2000 to 14 March 2001

Brain power

When one is nearing the last days of in-patient therapy, weekend jaunts home became routine. Any thoughts of what will be encountered are overshadowed by the fact that whatever is out there will be hopefully short lived. Returning to the safety of the hospital is imminent and was ever present in my mind. Some patients think that the final day signals the last of therapy and the next day everything will be back to normal as before their stroke. Of course, we know this couldn't be further from the truth as therapy is never over; its name is changed to at home frolics for the lack of a better name. Even on my last days after an extended therapy session, I had a comfortable feeling coupled with mixed emotions that my return for out-patient therapy in the coming weeks would allow for further improvements and contact with those who professionally guided me through this dilemma.

We were taught many other things during therapy; it was as if parts of my brain had become blank and had to be reprogrammed to do even the basics which were automatic before. Hospital routines were something that would be taken with me and remain deeply embedded, so much so that one did get somewhat annoyed should change be introduced or the routine interrupted. It is my opinion now, that the changes presented in the hospital only at a rate that each patient could recognize therefore, I had little problems there. At home, things were ever changing at a rate to fast for my brain. It kept playing catch up after the initial shock of outright confusion. My family was the first to identify these actions wondering if things would change down the road. In time, I too realized that broadening my horizons would and could be beneficial, now that my brain was functioning with increased capacity. By deliberately changing routines it has helped to get away from this tunnel vision of the mind but there still is some distance to go.

The weekly sessions of out-patient therapy proved to be very beneficial and I was extremely glad to have been offered this extra time. The hands-on therapy was basically the same even some mechanical devises were employed but the continuation allowed more improvement in muscle tone and endurance. Arriving in my brand new wheelchair, wheelchair you say! Why? Well, although I could walk short distances using only a cane by this time, I still wasn't equipped for those longer walks. Trips to the malls, barber shop and hospital were accomplished via the chair and it became a permanent fixture in the rear of our van. Eventually, it was used less and less until it became a conversation piece in our recreation room and on standby should it ever be needed again.

Deviating a bit from the stroke topic, I want to relay an important incident that happened on one of my later weekend's at home. After travelling at very slow wheelchair speeds in the hospital, the trips home with my wife driving; it seemed that she was practicing for the Indy 500. Initially, keeping my eyes closed or on the speedometer, I kept thinking of automobile insurance.

Reading the policy it was determined that I was obliged to notify the company of anything that might impair my driving abilities. Now being a law abiding citizen and knowing that the doctor in the hospital was obliged to inform the Ministry of Transport of Ontario of my stroke and told me not to drive, I called the insurance company and reported my condition. They informed me that they wouldn't cancel the insurance but would take my name off the policy and make my wife the principal driver. I had to sign a document indicating that I wouldn't drive which arrived in the mail two days later. Doing as they suggested, the document was faxed back which completed the transaction. In no way, am I suggesting everybody do this, however you should read your insurance policy very carefully to ensure its content. I was glad I did and you'll see why when we get to the driver examination part.

Soon I was saying goodbye to the out-patient therapist so that some other deserving individuals could get the same benefits as I did. Brain power kept increasing during this time frame however the left arm remained an ornament by my side. The doctors had said this would be the last to come back so it made one wonder if the doctors thought implant was impeding its return. That thought was erased one day during a conversation with my wife. You see I had unknowingly entered into the stroke survivor's world of "*no can do*" where the left arm was concerned. During the conversation she suggested, "that I should maybe try placing more emphasis on training it and start the exercise program sent home with me from the out-patient therapist". These included: elbow, forearm, shoulder, scapula, wrist and finger exercises. One for the upper body portion which seemed easy at first was to cross you arms across the chest and cup both elbows in the palm of your hands. With a rocking motion, as if rocking a baby, go back and forth from side to side about twenty-five times extending the arms outwards to the left and right as far as possible. As you commence this exercise the back, neck and shoulder muscles will sit up and take notice so don't over do it but stay the course each day. Now Mr. Procrastinator's holiday was about to end and for good reason. Practicing what I had been preaching to other patients at first became extremely difficult and the routine became intermittent however, self discipline eventually prevailed. Great results followed.

Two hands vs. one

The word *"Tried"* rattled around this old noggin for the next few hours until it finally sunk in that I had done very little to train my left arm to be something other than a filler for my shirt sleeve. I also realized that it was automatic to say, "I can't do that" without even thinking of trying. So this exercise proved to me that if you haven't tried to do something, how do you know you can or can't accomplish the task presented? From that day forth, I slowly attempted to involve the left arm as much as possible. The right arm did everything up to this point but it was beginning to show the wear and tear especially with the arthritis becoming more evident. On the other hand, the stroke delayed the arthritic progress but engaging it more, the arthritis is now playing catch up.

At this point my both little fingers were deformed and had repositioned themselves outwards to be caught on everything that came close. Putting ones hand in pockets was most annoying and almost impossible due to the out stretched pinky. A trip to a rheumatoid arthritic specialist concluded that a trip to a surgeon was warranted to see if corrective surgery could fix the problem. If not than amputation could be an alternative. My response to the latter was of course negative indicating that one came into this world with eight fingers and one would leave having the same. Sometime later relaying this story to my out patient therapist she looked the situation over and recommended that I grasp the wrist of the other arm or something of similar size and squeeze using all fingers holding this position for the count of five. Releasing the pressure then repeating the exercise about ten times per hand. This suggestion has produced excellent results; my both little fingers are no longer heading east and west as before, they are controllable and can again be put into pockets without catching the sides.

Some places where the left arm now assists include; the holding of a tilted breakfast bowl so that the last remaining cereal and milk could be retrieved. The holding of a dinner plate while scrapping off the scraps with the right or holding a bottle so the right can remove the top. Signing papers or documents using one hand is almost impossible so it was nice when the left hand could hold the paper even if it is placed there by the right. I haven't mastered those pesky plastic cereal bags that are inside the boxes so this is where help is required or the help of scissors to do the job. Another area attempted successfully was the drying after my shower. Thought it would be nice to have the towel around my back, this way I could dry my hair plus the back with a see-saw motion. Placing the towel around my neck I grasp it with both hands, one at each end with the left hand being placed first. The sawing motion did the trick to my enjoyment. Doing up shirt buttons was accomplished by laying on the bed for the top ones, this way the arm could remain horizontal. The bottom buttons were done up sitting up. To a family member or a non-stroke person these events are routine however, I can tell you they are pebbles along the rocky road of life which have turned into big boulders after a stroke. Conquering these identify success, progress and are milestones in the life of many stroke survivors.

One of the hardest movements to accomplish is that of getting the left arm up so you reach your mouth. Eating corn-on-the-cob poses a real problem and could only be accomplished if you had a neck like a cat. Seems the hand grip is strongest but the arm muscles fall short. This is bad enough for right handed people but must be devastating to lefties. Times like this you wish everyone could be ambidextrous. Speaking of grips, when working around the kitchen it's best to have some help if you like unsliced crusty bread. My first attempts ended up with the large part of the loaf being held by my left hand resembling that of bread pudding. Seems the grip control went south and is the hardest to control under all circumstances. In the grocery store, placing the left hand on the cart handle, one would have to fight to remove it to retrieve something off the shelves. Talking to it never helped, but on several occasions people wondered who I was talking to.

Not having mentioned much about the behavior of my left leg and foot so far it just sort of tagged along with the rest of my body's functions and only complaining if stubbed on the carpet or raised doorway. Now that the arm retraining program was underway, let's include the left leg and foot also. Its training started by the downwards pointing the toes for entry into shoes or slippers. Previously I had exercised the foot as my therapist suggested, bending the toes forward with great success. Once that was accomplished the next exercise was to rock the foot first lifting the toes as high as possible then the heel. Sounds like a dance, heel and toe. Many attempts failed but eventually the continued persistence paid off. Next would be the putting on of snow boots, this exercise included both leg, foot coordination plus hands and arms as well. The foot first had to be started into the boot then the both hands grasped high toppers to finish. Thanks to the makers of Velcro, securing the footwear is made easier. Everything should have Velcro closures on them. Not such an easy task but through time one successfully accomplished the job with great effort.

Butt muscles played a huge factor with the lower extremities. To strength them my exercise was to face my bedroom high boy or something of similar height placing both hands on the top with one foot slightly ahead of the other. Now tightening the butt, raise both feet so standing on tip toes, hold for the count of five and relax coming back to the standing position. After fifteen of these change foot positions with the other ahead and repeat the exercise another fifteen times. Talk about buns of steel this is how to achieve them plus it also helps with balance. While resting two thoughts always crossed my mind as the wind howled and the snow fell, wonder what the temperature is in Myrtle Beach, SC and why are we not there.

Mind and driver training

M ulti tasking had become a thing of the passed. There was a time when one could line up a dozen or so things to do. Well, would you believe a half dozen? Then prioritize and complete them to everyone's satisfaction. Now three or less topics overloaded the brain cells; the first you may complete, the second may be started, but the third drifted off into the sunset. This is very disturbing to people who use to be active and on the go. Training here proved to be much more complex as it was harder to track the progression, out of sight out of mind so to speak. To again be productive one had to clear all thoughts then plan or develop a technique to accomplish each task individually. This wasn't only true for extra duties but for everything including daily tasks such as morning showering, dressing etc. I was quite fortunate and it has been suggested that possibly my years of Air force training and employment may have aided in the faster recovery. For years we had been schooled in the factors that caused resistance to change in people, to the point where we did not always like the change but automatically accepted it until it was field tested and proven. Recently having read where it was found that the left and right sides of the brain interact with each other, this may have also accelerated the tasking and thought process.

As time passed, improvements all around continued at their own pace. The amount of effort put in reaped the rewards, to a point, but yet again things were slow. This sure dispelled one myth from outside the stroke rehabilitation world, which was that at the one year anniversary that would be as good as it gets. No more improvements what-so-ever. Bull Pucky!

Never having any desire to this point to get behind the wheel of our van and drive, the thought occurred to me that maybe I should do some pre-study in case the urge came to me. My daughter picked up a copy of the "Rules of the Road" and I proceeded to refresh my memory. One surprising fact came to mind as I was reading each section; my mind was accepting the numerous facts listed within, with very little overload. Was this total recall? Happy that this was so, I was also aware that exploring all these driving situations was done on the safety of the living room couch. Out in the real world things would be much different. Studying completed to my satisfaction I still was apprehensive of what lay ahead. The hospital had applied to the Ottawa Rehabilitation Centre for me to be evaluated for driving, however, no word had been received. It wasn't until one afternoon, my wife and I were having a cup of coffee in the living room when she made the statement that "Your back"! Asking for an explanation because I did not think I went anywhere, she informed me that I was now thinking and talking much like before the stroke. This came as quite a shock but sure made me feel good. So much so, that I proceeded a few days later to our van to sit in the driver's seat and evaluate what could or couldn't be done.

Turning and viewing out the side windows posed no problems, the back windows were the same applying a little more attention. The rear and side view mirrors were also engaged successfully, with the understanding of what was being viewed. My left foot maintained positions away from under the brake peddle and its position was known at all times. Evaluating the left hand possibilities proved very little could be done with it, at this point, but the promise was made that every effort to someday reach the light, signal and windshield switches and turn them on and off would be accomplished. In the meantime, I was aware of aides were available to assist these situations should I be successful through the driving evaluation. A bar to be attached to the turning signal lever to reverse its operation to the right side was available. Also a spinner knob placed on the steering wheel would assist in the steering of the van and make it easier especially in tight spaces. All-in-all the van exploration was positive as was the studying so now the confidence level was reaching a new high. Was I ready? We all thought so.

The Rehabilitation Centre was contacted only to find that the application sent to them by the hospital never arrived or at least my name wasn't in their computer. For a stroke survivor really wanting to drive, *Panic!* This was short lived however, as they found that it was sent and due to the two year plus time frame I would be accepted soonest. Now this was Friday so how about Tuesday? *Panic!* My brain overload light flickered but only for a second. Settling myself down, I accepted the appointment and immediately after getting off the phone called the optometrist office for a peripheral vision test which had to be provided during the testing for my records. Next, Para Transpo had to be contacted for a ride there and back on the designated days. Things were now progressing which was good, would they stay that way? Time would tell.

Driving evaluation

Holding my peripheral vision test results and a letter of authenticity the trip was under way to the Ottawa Rehab. Centre. Gazing out the window of the Para Transpo vehicle, I wondered what was in store and how would I cope. The studying had been completed, my mind identified its readiness and there was a complete calmness assuring me all would be OK. The later came about after I evaluated the situation and told myself that attempts are made and without them nothing is gained. Also the two million or so accident free miles that I've accumulated meant very little and should not even be considered. Failure was always a possibility but it wasn't a positive so be gone with it.

Arriving there I was registered and ushered into a large class type room where the proceedings started. First I was positioned in front of and centered at a long board housing a single row of lights on each side. Looking directly at a spot I was requested to indicate which side the lights came on, left or right. Next, we discussed some rules of the road using road, intersection diagrams plus other questions pertaining to driving skills. Lastly, in a mock-up of a vehicle driver's compartment complete with brake, gas peddle, console and lights, steering wheel etc.

I began testing. Reflex action came first, red light hit the brake and green light back to the gas peddle. At this point I was asked if my left foot posed any problem and if I knew where it was all the time. They wanted to make sure that it wasn't under the brake peddle impeding the brakes action which it wasn't. Next a film was run on a screen ahead of the mock-up indicating some streets and road ways in San Francisco. Studying the movie the realism was fantastic. Heavy traffic, multi-lanes both straight and turning, traffic lights, stop signs, the works was presented. There was even a basket ball bouncing across the road and I was there in the midst of it all. This exercise provided life like challenges throughout but it was a real confidence builder. No pedestrians were run over or fenders bent, no red lights gone through or speed limits exceeded. The rules of the road were observed and successfully completed, another milestone accomplished.

As the day progressed, it was discovered that my driver license had not been suspended so we were taken for a quite residential drive in a Driver's Education car, with me driving. Quickly, it was determined that my left hand was ineffective so a spinner knob plus a turn signal bar was installed for my use. This made things easier however the final analysis at the end of the trial was that I needed a couple of driving lessons. Scheduling and completing these two outing afforded me the opportunity to become more familiar with a car rather than the van I had been driving before. I was picked up at home and returned there on each occasion. That finished, the final testing was done in centre town and on the busiest of Ottawa's highways. Returning to the rehab centre the evaluation complete, I was told that a passing grade had been achieved so good luck in my future driving. With that, the therapist passed me a work order to get our van equipped with the instruments needed and suggested that the paperwork would be relayed to the Ministry of Transport of Ontario (MTO) at Toronto in the coming days.

Remember the part about me calling my insurance company and identifying my condition, they in turn made my wife the principal driver removing my name from the policy. Now I hoped it was the time to reverse this situation. Arriving home on my last Para Transpo run I called my insurance company and informed them that I had completed the driver evaluation and that I was good to go, however, no driving would be accomplished until my insurance coverage was reinstated.

The agent asked me to 'please hold until the underwriters could be contacted'. A few minutes later he returned to inform me 'that as of this moment I was fully covered with no increase in premiums'. 'No paperwork required' I asked, 'No you were honest with us so we are returning the favor, have a great day and an insert renaming you as principal driver should arrive in the mail within a few days'. What a relief! Sure pays to be honest, say what!

The next day arrangements were made for the equipment to be installed in our van. Upon completion the renewed sense of freedom was overwhelming. I felt like a 16 year old kid again on a joy ride. Another milestone, another accomplishment and hopes for more yet to come. The new found joy went on for about thirty days when a letter came from MTO Toronto suggesting that due to a report received it was identified that I may have problems driving my vehicle. To dispel any so-called problems I would have to take the MTO drivers test complete with written, eye exam and road test within 30 days or my license would be cancelled. Was the wind knocked out of my sails, only for a moment or two, because the prior evaluation prepared me for any testing requirement?

My promise to return

Attempting to determine the reason MTO came to the conclusion that I may have trouble driving our van remains a mystery even today. Getting no where during a conversation with the letter's editor, I thanked the gentleman from Toronto for his time and dialed our licensing establishment here in Ottawa. Arrangements were made and the eye test plus written was accomplished in one sitting. The on-road driving test was slated five days later and preceded without a huge hitch. After returning to the bureau's parking lot, the examiner identified that I had passed however, I had made many mistakes. Citing the first part of her statement, I requested that she sign the paper and pass it to me. This being finished I now was ready to discuss the last part of her statement. We talked, discussed but never argued. I learned of all my bad driving habits which were imbedded over the years but did get in the last words. "Thank you, Madam".

The winter months came upon us and I curtailed some of my driving activity. The sunny days were inviting but the cold biting wind kept me indoors on most days. My measurement for cold came when I saw a dog chasing a cat and they were both walking, that was to cold. Of course, Grumpies taxi and shuttle service still operated when the family outings dictated a must go situation. In late winter, early spring of 2004, the driving bug hit again. The snow was going down and the promise I had made to the good Lord that I would return to the stroke ward was now a real possibility. He had allowed me to become mobile on my own and the patients could stand some encouragement from a survivor who had gone through the whole gambit.

Contacting our previous social worker it was found out that stroke ward ID of St. Vincent had moved to the 4th floor of Elisabeth Bruyere, complete with staffing. This was welcomed news as the much more acquired space was realized with the relocation. She also informed me of a new development that had been directed by one of the Recreational Therapists. That was the initiation of a coffee pot for inpatients, occurring every Wednesday afternoon. Patients could gather away from therapy, evaluations and their rooms to meet other patients and discuss daily topics of their choice. Two stroke survivors had already volunteered to assist in the operation but maybe one more would be welcome. Making contact with the Recreational Therapist, she outlined her thoughts on the program. The more I heard about it and the more involved, the more enthusiastic I became. Soon, I was introduce to the Volunteer Coordinator where the indoctrinations commenced and I became a full fledge Bruyere Volunteer.

Other aspirations and dreams

Stroke wise, my wife and I still had many aspirations; one was to visit the Maritimes where we had spent so much of our lives. Could this be done in my condition? The only way to prove that it could or couldn't was to try. Packing up the van, we headed out driving some 3400 kilometers visiting: New Brunswick for some good lobsters dinners; staying in a chalet on Cape Breton Island for a week plus visiting with our long time Myrtle Beach friends in Sydney; then to the south eastern shore of Nova Scotia to Mahone Bay for another week in a chalet; heading down to Yarmouth, NS we visited with some other friends; crossing to the Annapolis Valley, we headed north east and took a trip across the new Confederation Bridge to Prince Edward Island just to say we had crossed it. On to St John, NB and home through the upper states stopping for some good Vermont maple butter and syrup.

Problems occurred along the way but nothing one couldn't handle with help of a loving wife. Driving was done by me, making sure we were off the road fairly early or when I started to get tired. Frequent stops at rest areas to stretch the legs helped with the routine of the longer drives. In motels and chalets showering posed a small problem as the showers were inside the tub enclosures. To remedy this situation one sat on the edge of the tub and placed each foot one at a time inside on the non-skid tub floor then standing with the help of a faucet or tap. To get out the reverse was employed without incident or accident.

All and all the trip proved the possibility existed that we could travel and enjoy the pleasures afforded us before my stroke, other thoughts included perhaps returning to the warmer climate of Myrtle Beach, SC for a few weeks during the cold winters of Ottawa. This too was accomplished for two years with the hope to returning again however, the passing of our friend's wife that vacationed with us and my wife of 50 years, 3 months and 13 days (27 May 2009) both taken by cancer has curtailed this event.

Positive vs. negative

The text so far has been nothing but positive because I am a positive sort of guy or a least that's what I understood until falling into the human trap. This segment is included not to discourage but to inform, so that the reader whoever he or she may be is aware the unthinkable can happen without warning to the best of us. In my case, the letting go of my in-house physiotherapist the trip preparation commence for our second retreat to the good old USA to get away from the harsh winter and cold weather. The call of the south was again overwhelming and the distraction completely changed my routine, so much so that all exercises pretty much went out the door. Packing suit cases, dragging them do to the van and loading them justified in my mind that enough was done for this body to survive. Driving those long hours further justified no workouts today or the next and the next until we arrived at our destination. Did I feel guilty for changing the habits that helped me maintain a state of wellness? Not on your life because my mind told me everything had been justified and the right thing was happening. *Wrong!*

R & R (Rest and Relaxation) became the order of the day watching for dolphins swimming by and as if watching

TV at home the snacks and drinks were close by and consumed on a regular basis. Dinners were a must outside the condo visiting one specialty house after another each night for Texas steak, King crab legs etc. Party time all the time!

As time elapsed the return home did nothing for my forgotten exercise routine as the same justification for not doing it remained the same. A somewhat different routine was adopted with the same old excuses; this time justifying the many taxi runs taking the granddaughters, their friends and other family members to their various sporting and shopping activities was deemed ample activity. *Wrong!*

The total disregard I had for my body began to take its toll, energy was diminished, get up and go got up and went and worst of all my being glucose intolerant was now heading for full blown diabetes. You see that important function of timely readings also went by the wayside. Wake up call? Well I guess! The irony of it all, for months I had been in a developed routine produced by the experts and if not getting better by leaps and bounds, I was maintaining a life style that was acceptable and cherishing every minute of it. Also, I had set a double standard for the first time in my life telling other stroke survivors that the rehabilitation doesn't stop the day you leave the hospital program; it is forever so please continue with those important exercises and stay the course.

Bruyere coffee pot

Within Bruyere, this place of healing, the staff members can only be called "the beautiful people". Their inner beauty is projected to each patient and in turn grasped upon by them at a time when most vulnerable. As a means of regaining self exposure a recreation therapist re-established and expanded an event that was named "the coffee pot" and did so with the idea to give the stroke in-patients a meeting place away from the clinical atmosphere. They could get out of their rooms and away from the scrutiny of the continuous evaluations. It was to be a place to unwind before or after therapy of all kinds and could be visited alone or accompanied by their families or close friends. Also it was to be a collecting place to meet other patients and discuss mutual things of interest or just get to know each other. Another benefit the therapist thought would be an advantage was to recruit stroke survivors into the team. These volunteers would have gone through the rehabilitation process and could explain their experiences and encourage those presently in-house. Having this process started on a weekly basis, she, in no way could ever realize the full potential that would be evident in the near or distant future but hoped it would be successful.

Automatically it became a tremendous success! Patients and families alike attended on a regular basis not wanting to miss out on the excellent coffee, conversation and companionship. Out-patients returning for therapy all wanted their therapy to fall on the Wednesday to coincide with the coffee pot but unfortunately only a few spaces where available. Therapists from all departments used the gathering to further their patients involvement, bringing them at the end of their regular sessions and dropping them off so they could tell of their plight and be reassured by others of their progress, most of which they were unaware. Successful indeed, the coffee pot became a regular gathering place for more than in-patients; it was visited regularly by former patients so that in-patients were finding difficulty attending due to the crowd. At this point other agencies were approach to find spaces to accommodate the large number.

Topics of conversations around the table often include benefits patients can apprise themselves of such as T2201, Disability tax credit where they can receive a break on their income tax. Submissions can be done at any point as the date of the stroke is the commencement of benefit, if qualified. One note; the patient or family member should produce a rough draft of each section they qualify in as their family doctors probably hasn't seen them or know their limitations and conversations are soon forgotten. Handicap parking passes is another topic often discussed complete with the city bylaws governing same. Periodically some versed in piano playing will sit down and serenade the group. One such case, two people with different effected sides teamed up with each playing with their good side. This twosome melded together as one and enjoyed by all.

The aquatic exercise programs available at various locations around the city and attended by the recreation therapist are discussed for those approaching the end of rehabilitation and would like to participate further with supervised conditioning. On the lighter side; many would be comics emerge and stories are told of grandchildren, like the one who was going to be a professional basketball player when he grew up as he was dribbling all over the place now. Many tales have been told of lifetime experiences, most bring smiles to those present and for that instant they are taken away from the lows of that emotional rollercoaster. Frowns and ever tears have been changed to smiles or laughter and this means a lot to the volunteers and therapists, we have accomplished something meaningful and often lasting. Some encounters with patients or family members were a real challenge even for this stroke survivor. On one occasion a family member arrived at the coffee pot awaiting her husband to complete his round of therapy with a very disgruntled look Sitting by herself I approached saying, "your not yourself today, is there anything you would like to discuss". Turning towards me with tears in her eyes she said "she had just been informed that her husband was going to be an invalid for the rest of his life". *Say what?* Now knowing her husband and his progress to date I was totally confused due to the fact that just last week I asked him "when he was going to get that wheelchair off his butt" which he replied "soon I hope". Could something have happened that I was yet unaware of? Really puzzled and taken aback as I could not remember anyone of hospital staff using that type of terminology. Continuing the conversation and hoping not to offend her I asked "exactly what was said to you"? "Well", "we were at a family conference this morning and they told me to go out and purchase a wheelchair for my husband". A sigh of relief engulfed me but was minor as to her immediate reactions when I told her that that was standard operating procedure and that mine was still in the back of my van in case travel distance for shopping was know to be to far then it would be used by me to complete the required distance. Her relief was overwhelming and the remained of her stay was much more pleasant especially when she saw her husband entering the room out of his wheelchair and pushing a walker. His first comment was, "look John, I got the wheelchair off my butt"! This term has remained throughout the weeks that followed and is only used by the stroke survivors should one get the feeling that the patient has become complacent and unwilling to try to walk.

Many wonderful stories have been told around the table and we encourage every patient and family members to attend the coffee pot, come on down, please enjoy the coffee and goodies provided, the only charge is a smile.

As of March 2010, it will be my 6 year anniversary being involved with the coffee pot, over three of those years my wife Margaret baked muffins, squares and other goodies for the patients. We both realized a most rewarding experience, her with the written and verbal accolades received from patients and staff alike, mine by the witnessing of the repeated weekly improvements of the patients. This, at first may only be a slight movement of an affected arm or leg; a word or two uttered; a sparkle in the eye or a major change of a wheelchair for a walker or cane. These rewards are unequalled and payment beyond belief. Each week when I return home and relay the days happenings to my family we marvel at the progress of the patients and many times have concluded that we wished a coffee pot had of been available when we were going through our ordeal.

Ten years later

As time passed more contacts were made out in the stroke community. The Stroke Survivors Association of Ottawa was one of the organizations that caught my interest as they were providing stroke patients in the area with important information and assistance during and after rehabilitation, much the same as we were doing in the Bruyere hospitals stroke ward. Their Peer- to-Peer program provided visitations to hospital wards on a regular basis to encourage stroke patient through therapy, and to inform them as to what services were available in the community and to ensure them that they had a friendly contact to call when discharged from the hospital should they so desire.

Attending one of the board meetings to find out more of their organization I was told that a board position, that of Vice Chairman, had come available and they were looking for someone with my experience to fill it. Talk about timing or was this planned? It really didn't matter as I had read and heard enough to this point about all their good work that acceptance of the position was automatic. Since that evening collectively, we have embarked on further programs to enhance the awareness and participation not only inside to community but outside as well. The formation of a Peer-to-Peer group in Pembroke, north of Ottawa has been started and it is the intent to organize similar out laying communities the same guidance during their set up process.

Another tasking that is underway is that of a Living with Stroke program to be taught in our community with the instructors all being stroke survivors themselves. The course is offered to stroke patients and their care givers, with the care giver attending and participating as one half of their team. Also, as the name implies, it is to equip both to better understand and cope with the struggles that lay ahead.

Thank you St. Vincent, Bruyere, and the Stroke Survivors Association for all that you do and have done. Thank you for all the individuals within these organizations that make it happen. Some day, maybe not in this lifetime, your just reward will be realized and you will be credited for your compassion, caring, understanding, dedication and professionalism revealed to those stroke patients at the time when most vulnerable and in desperate need.

Now that my account is drawing to a close hopefully, I have accomplished the goal initially set out, which was to explain what an individual goes through after having a stroke. With a bit of luck someone, whether a stroke survivor, care giver, family member or a friend will get some comfort and a better understanding of stroke from reading this book. Resulting in the realization as I, that stroke patients need the everlasting love of family and friends and most important come to the conclusion there *is life after stroke* and it's worth fighting and conquering the hardships along the way.

Good Luck to all survivors and may God bless everyone!